BENEATH THE SURFACE

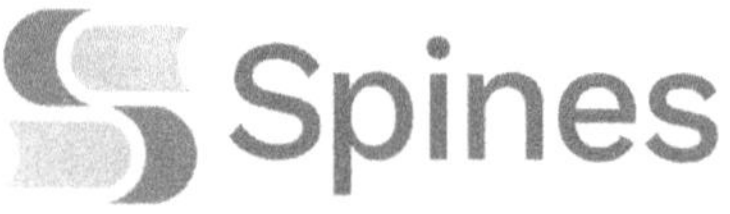
Spines

BENEATH THE SURFACE

UNRAVELING THE MYSTERIES OF ALOPECIA

ALICIA BAKER

ACKNOWLEDGMENTS

First, I would like to thank my Lord and Savior for all of my blessings. Writing this book wouldn't have been possible without putting GOD first in my life.

AMEN!

For My Children,

Lamarra R Jones, thank you for always being there to give me advice on all of my endeavors and accomplishments. You have inspired me to continue to educate people on the types of alopecia and its causes.

Spenser M Baker, thank you for your kind words, and questions about hair follicles and hair growth. Your questions gave me insight on writing this book about alopecia and its causes.

For my Siblings,

I love you all and thank you for sharing your thoughts, ideas and time and always being there in more ways than one.

To Rhonda V. Johnson, thank you for giving me advice and being humorous during the times that I really needed it. To Tyheisha S. Wright, thank you for being yourself and sharing your encouraging and inspirational words. To Ronald V. Forehand, thank you for always being there and giving me encouragement on my successes. To Anthony R Morris, thank you for traveling to Florida with me to get my Trichology degree and giving me lots of encouragement on my successes. To Ronald V Morris, thank you for always being there with your encouraging words. To James A Morris, thank you for lending me your ear when I needed to talk about my present and future business ventures.

Thank you to all.

Your mom, and sister

Alicia.

CONTENTS

INTRODUCTION

Alopecia, often perceived as a mere aesthetic concern, transcends superficial distress, embedding itself into the lives of those it touches with profound psychological and emotional implications. This book aims to demystify alopecia by providing a comprehensive overview of what the condition entails, its causes, and the various treatment options available. In an effort to bridge the gap between scientific jargon and accessible understanding, our journey through these pages will be guided by empathy, clarity, and an unwavering focus on offering support and empowerment to those navigating this condition.

The term "alopecia" itself might sound technical, yet it embodies a wide spectrum of experiences characterized by hair loss. The condition does not discriminate, affecting individuals across all demographics. However, the impact and the way it is perceived can vary dramatically from one person to another. Our exploration begins with a foundation of understanding, breaking down the basics of alopecia, its different types, and how they manifest in individuals. This foundational knowledge is crucial for anyone looking to grasp the nature of their condition or to empathize with those experiencing it.

Recognizing the symptoms of alopecia and understanding when to seek medical advice are pivotal steps in the journey towards managing this condition. Early detection and consultation with a healthcare provider can dramatically influence the effectiveness of the treatment plan. However, identifying the symptoms can be a challenge in itself, given the natural variability in hair growth and loss among individuals. This book aims to clarify these symptoms, offering a guideline for when professional advice should be sought.

Diagnosis of alopecia can feel like a turning point in one's journey. It confirms the presence of the condition but also heralds the start of a new chapter filled with questions about what comes next. This book delves into the diagnostic approaches used by healthcare professionals, the tools and tests that play a critical role in determining the type of alopecia, and the most appropriate treatment paths moving forward.

Understanding the underlying causes of alopecia is not just about satisfying scientific curiosity; it's about providing comfort and context to those affected. By exploring genetic factors and environmental triggers, this book sheds light on why alopecia occurs, dispelling myths, and grounding the discussion in verifiable evidence. This understanding is crucial in mitigating the condition's psychological toll, offering a semblance of control and predictability in an otherwise uncertain journey.

The emotional and psychological dimensions of dealing with alopecia cannot be overstated. Fear, anxiety, and a hit to one's self-esteem are common companions along this path. However, this book aims not only to acknowledge these feelings but also to offer strategies for building resilience, confidence, and ultimately, a path towards emotional well-being. By addressing these aspects, we ensure a holistic approach to managing alopecia, emphasizing the importance of mental health in the overall treatment plan.

Treatment options for alopecia are as varied as the condition itself, encompassing everything from medications and topical solutions to alternative therapies. The role of diet and nutritional choices also garners significant attention, underlining the interconnectedness of lifestyle factors and hair health. This book will sift through these various treatment options, providing a balanced view of what works, what doesn't, and where the jury is still out.

Our exploration is not limited to the confines of Western medicine alone. Alopecia is a global condition, and as such, cultural insights and international approaches to treatment offer invaluable perspectives. By embracing a broad view, readers can appreciate the diverse ways in which different cultures tackle alopecia, enriching the tapestry of solutions and coping mechanisms available.

As we embark on this journey together, it's important to remember that the road to understanding and managing alopecia is not always straightforward. But with each chapter, our goal is to equip you with knowledge, understanding, and hope. Through the amalgamation of scientific insights, empathetic guidance, and practical advice, this book strives to be a companion and a resource for anyone looking to navigate the challenges of alopecia.

In essence, this book is more than a collection of information; it's an enormous amount of support, designed to stand by you, illuminate the path ahead, and help you make informed decisions about your health and well-being. Welcome to a resource crafted to help you understand alopecia in all its dimensions – let's take this step towards understanding and empowerment together.

CHAPTER 1
ALOPECIA: AN OVERVIEW

ALOPECIA ISN'T JUST A CONDITION; IT'S A JOURNEY THAT many unexpectedly find themselves on, navigating through complex emotions, varying symptoms, and a sea of treatments. At its core, alopecia is the medical term for hair loss, a seemingly simple definition that barely scratches the surface of this multifaceted issue. While we're about to dive deep into its basics, including its types and how they manifest, it's crucial to understand that this chapter sets the stage for a more comprehensive exploration. Hair loss can affect anyone, regardless of age or gender, and its impact is not solely physical. The subsequent chapters will delve into recognizing signs, understanding causes, and exploring both medical and alternative treatments. Furthermore, we'll examine the psychological effects of alopecia and ways to mitigate them, highlighting the importance of mental well-being in this journey. Remember, while alopecia may be challenging, understanding its nuances is the first step toward empowerment and, ultimately, finding a path that's right for you.

Understanding the Basics

Alopecia, a term that might sound esoteric at first mention, is essentially the medical term for hair loss, a condition that affects millions of people worldwide. Before we dive deep into its complexities, it's crucial to lay the groundwork by first understanding what alopecia isn't. It's not a sign of severe sickness, nor is it contagious. However, its impact extends beyond the physical aspect, often touching the emotional and psychological well-being of those affected.

The causes of alopecia are varied and often complex. While we'll delve into the specifics in later sections, it's important at this juncture to acknowledge that alopecia can stem from multiple factors. These range from genetic predispositions to environmental triggers such as stress, diet, and even certain medications. Learning about these causes not only helps in demystifying alopecia but also sets the stage for a better understanding of potential treatments and management strategies.

Treatment for alopecia is as varied as its causes, encompassing a vast array of options from medical interventions to natural remedies and lifestyle modifications. While the prospect of navigating through these options can seem daunting at first, knowledge is a powerful tool in making informed decisions. It's through understanding the basics that individuals can start to discern which steps to take next, guided not by fear or misinformation but by facts and professional advice.

Understanding alopecia also means recognizing its unpredictable nature. The condition can manifest in different ways, ranging from small, unnoticeable patches to complete loss of hair on the scalp or even the entire body. This variability underscores the importance of early diagnosis and personalized treatment plans. It's a journey that is unique for everyone, with successes, setbacks, and everything in between.

As we move forward, keep in mind that while alopecia may be a part of someone's life, it doesn't define them. The journey through understanding, managing, and living with alopecia is one of resilience, hope, and discovery. By starting with the basics, we lay a strong foundation for not just coping with alopecia but thriving in spite of it.

What Is Alopecia?

Alopecia is a condition that might sound foreign but is far more common than many think. In its essence, alopecia is the medical term for hair loss, a condition affecting millions worldwide regardless of age or gender. It's not just about finding a few strands of hair on your pillow in the morning; this condition can lead to significant hair loss on the scalp and, in some cases, the entire body. Alopecia is not discriminatory; it can strike anyone at any stage of life, causing more than just physical changes—it can also deeply impact an individual's psychological state and social interactions.

At its core, alopecia is categorized into several types, but before diving into the complexities, it's crucial to understand the fundamental nature of this condition. The human hair cycle consists of growth, rest, and shedding phases. When this cycle is disrupted, either by genetics, medical conditions, or other factors, alopecia can occur. The disruption leads to noticeable hair loss, which can range from small patches to complete baldness.

The reasons behind alopecia are as varied as the individuals it affects. From autoimmune responses where the body attacks its own hair follicles, thinking them to be foreign, to genetic predispositions that make one more susceptible to hair loss. Stress, certain medications, and underlying health conditions can also play significant roles in the development of alopecia. It's a complex tapestry of causes that requires a thorough understanding to address effectively.

Treatment for alopecia depends largely on its type and

the underlying cause. While some types of alopecia might be temporary and the hair can grow back, others may result in permanent hair loss. Currently, there are treatments available that can help slow down the process or stimulate hair growth, such as medication, laser therapy, or even surgical options like hair transplants. However, the effectiveness of these treatments varies from person to person, and addressing the psychological impact is also a critical component of managing alopecia.

Understanding alopecia involves recognizing it as more than just a superficial issue. It's a complex condition that can deeply affect one's self-esteem and quality of life. Awareness and education on the matter can help pave the way for empathy, support, and more effective solutions for those coping with this condition. It's about looking beyond the hair loss and seeing the individual, providing them with the necessary tools to navigate the challenges alopecia brings into their lives.

Types of Alopecia

Alopecia, a condition that can lead to hair loss on the scalp and other parts of the body, manifests in various forms, each with unique characteristics and implications for those affected. Understanding the different types of alopecia is crucial for comprehending this complex condition, its causes, and the potential treatments available. This section delves into the main categories and subtypes of alopecia, providing insights into their distinct features.

Alopecia Areata

Is an autoimmune condition where the immune system mistakenly attacks hair follicles, leading to hair loss. This type of alopecia typically results in one or more small, round patches of baldness on the scalp, but it can also affect other areas of the body. Alopecia areata can progress into more severe forms, such as alopecia totalis, where all scalp hair is lost, or alopecia universalis, resulting in the loss of all body hair.

Androgenetic Alopecia

Commonly known as male or female pattern hair loss, is characterized by a gradual thinning of hair, which often leads to partial or complete baldness. In men, this typically starts with a receding hairline and thinning on the crown, while women usually experience a broadening of the part in their hair. This form of alopecia is largely attributed to genetic predisposition and hormonal changes.

Telogen Effluvium

Represents a temporary form of alopecia where an abnormal number of hairs transition into the resting (telogen) phase of the hair growth cycle, leading to increased shedding. This condition can be triggered by severe stress, major surgery, childbirth, or severe illness. In most cases, telogen effluvium is reversible, with hair growth returning to normal within six months to a year.

Anagen Effluvium

Is predominantly caused by the interruption of the hair growth (anagen) phase, leading to widespread hair loss. This type is commonly associated with chemotherapy or radiation therapy but can also result from poisoning with toxic substances like arsenic or thallium. Anagen effluvium often occurs quite rapidly, within days or weeks of the damaging event.

Traction Alopecia

Results from persistent pulling or tension on hair strands over an extended period, commonly due to specific hairstyles (tight ponytails, braids, or dreadlocks) or the use of hair extensions. This mechanical stress leads to hair breakage and loss, primarily around the hairline and temples.

Central Centrifugal Cicatricial Alopecia (CCCA)

Is a type of scarring alopecia that primarily affects women of African descent, beginning at the crown of the scalp and progressing outward. This condition destroys hair follicles, replacing them with scar tissue and rendering the hair loss permanent. Early detection and intervention are crucial.

Frontal Fibrosing Alopecia

Presents as a receding hairline and thinning eyebrows, predominantly affecting postmenopausal women. The hair follicles are gradually replaced with scar tissue, leading to permanent hair loss. The exact causes of this condition remain unclear, but it's thought to involve hormonal and immune system components.

Lichen Planopilaris

Is a form of scarring alopecia where lichen planus, an inflammatory skin condition, affects the scalp. It results in patchy hair loss, redness, and scaling around hair follicles. The inflammation can permanently damage the hair follicles if not treated promptly.

Evidence suggests a connection between lifestyle factors and certain types of alopecia, such as diet's role in exacerbating or mitigating hair loss in cases of androgenetic alopecia. However, the effectiveness of lifestyle modifications can vary widely among individuals and types of alopecia.

Diagnosis of the specific type of alopecia typically involves a detailed medical history, physical examination, and may include scalp biopsies, blood tests, or other diagnostic tools to rule out underlying health issues and pinpoint the condition precisely. The exact approach will depend on the individual's symptoms and the suspected type of alopecia.

Treatment options for alopecia are as varied as the conditions themselves. They range from topical treatments and oral medications to light therapy and, in some cases, surgical options like hair transplantation. The choice of treatment is influenced by the type of alopecia, its severity, and the patient's preferences and overall health. Emerging therapies, including stem cell research and gene therapy, hold promise for future treatment pathways.

Living with alopecia can be challenging, not only physically but also emotionally. Those affected might grapple with issues of self-esteem and identity, underscoring the importance of a support network and professional psychological support in managing the condition. The psychological implications of alopecia, particularly those forms that lead to significant or total hair loss, can't be understated.

As research into alopecia advances, our understanding of this complex set of conditions continues to grow. This evolving comprehension helps to refine treatment strategies, offering hope to those affected by the various forms of alopecia. With ongoing support and advancements in treatment, many individuals with alopecia can manage their condition effectively, maintaining a high quality of life.

In closing, alopecia is more than just hair loss; it is a diverse group of conditions with a range of causes, manifestations, and treatment options. Understanding the types of alopecia is a crucial step for anyone looking to navigate the challenges it presents, whether they are facing the condition themselves or supporting someone who is. As we continue to learn more about alopecia, the potential for effective treatment and the support available to those affected only broadens, underscoring the importance of continued research and awareness in this field.

CHAPTER 2
THE SYMPTOMS OF ALOPECIA

IF YOU'RE ON A QUEST TO UNDERSTAND ALOPECIA, recognizing its symptoms is a fundamental step. Alopecia, in its various forms, doesn't always shout its presence from the rooftops. Instead, it might whisper through subtle changes, making it vital to pay attention to the clues our bodies provide. Let's concentrate on the signs that may indicate the onset of alopecia, understanding that awareness is the first step towards addressing the condition.

Alopecia's main symptom, regardless of its type, is hair loss. This can manifest differently depending on the individual and the specific form of alopecia they're experiencing. Some may find clumps of hair on their pillow upon waking, while others might notice gradual thinning when styling their hair or even abrupt bald patches that seem to appear overnight. It's important to recognize that hair loss isn't exclusively confined to the scalp; alopecia can affect any hair-bearing area of the body, making it a condition with a potentially wide-ranging impact on appearance and self-image.

Beyond hair loss, other symptoms can often go unnoticed or be misattributed to other causes. For instance, some individuals might experience itching or tingling sensations in areas where hair loss is about to occur. While these symptoms are less common, they can serve as early indicators of an underlying issue that merits attention. Similarly, noticing changes in the nails, such as pitting or roughness, could also be a clue, as alopecia and certain nail conditions are sometimes interconnected.

Given the varied nature of alopecia's presentation, it's understandable why someone might hesitate to seek medical advice, especially if the symptoms seem manageable or barely noticeable at first. However, timely consultation with a healthcare professional can provide clarity, not just in confirming the presence of alopecia but also in understanding its type and potential causes. This step is crucial for navigating the path towards effective management and treatment strategies.

Alopecia is not just a physical condition; it's a signal, a narrative of what's happening beneath the surface. Recognizing its symptoms is the beginning of a journey —a journey that might be challenging but is also filled with hope and possibilities for management and recovery. Like pieces of a puzzle, each symptom provides valuable insight, guiding us towards a better understanding of our bodies and the complexities of alopecia.

Recognizing the Signs

When it comes to identifying alopecia, spotting the initial signs is crucial. Typically, the most evident symptom is the unexpected loss of hair. This can manifest in various ways, ranging from small, round patches on the scalp to a more widespread thinning across the entire head. It's important to remember that hair loss can also occur on other parts of the body, such as the eyebrows, eyelashes, and facial hair. This might not always be as noticeable but can be just as significant a sign of alopecia.

Another sign to be aware of is significant hair shedding. Everyone sheds hair daily; it's a natural part of the hair's lifecycle. However, if you're finding large clumps of hair in your brush or shower drain regularly, it might be more than just the average shedding. This is especially concerning if the hair loss is accompanied by other symptoms, such as itching or burning sensations on the scalp, which can suggest underlying scalp conditions contributing to the hair loss.

Changes in the nails can also be an unexpected but telling symptom of certain types of alopecia, such as alopecia areata. These changes might include pitting, white spots, lines, and changes in texture. Though less common, these nail conditions are indicative of more systemic issues and should not be overlooked.

It's worth noting that the psychological impact of recognizing these signs should not be underestimated. The experience of losing hair can be distressing, leading to a significant emotional toll. Acknowledging the signs early and seeking emotional support is just as vital as addressing the physical symptoms. The sooner you can come to terms with these changes, the quicker you can start exploring the appropriate avenues for management and treatment.

Finally, while recognizing these signs is instrumental in identifying alopecia, self-diagnosis should not replace professional medical advice. If you're experiencing any of these symptoms, schedule a visit with a healthcare provider. The symptoms of alopecia can mimic those of other conditions, making an accurate diagnosis critical for effective treatment. Upcoming chapters will delve deeper into diagnostic approaches and treatments options, providing a comprehensive guide for managing alopecia at any stage.

When to Seek Medical Advice

Discovering sudden hair loss or finding bald patches on your scalp can understandably be a cause for concern. Recognizing when it's time to seek medical advice is critical not only for addressing alopecia but also for ruling out other possible health issues. If you notice an unusual amount of hair falling out during routine activities such as brushing or washing your hair, it may be time to consult a healthcare professional. It's particularly urgent if your hair loss is accompanied by other symptoms, such as itching, burning, or pain on your scalp.

Experiencing dramatic hair loss after a significant life event, such as childbirth, major surgery, or a severe illness, is not uncommon. While it's often temporary, reaching out to a doctor can provide peace of mind and treatment options to manage your symptoms more effectively. Moreover, if you start to notice patterns of hair loss that run in your family, seeking medical advice early on can help you understand your risk factors and potential genetic predisposition to alopecia.

Finding bald patches that rapidly increase in size or experiencing significant thinning over a short period can be indicative of an underlying condition that needs immediate attention. Certain types of alopecia, such as alopecia areata, can progress quickly, making timely intervention crucial. A healthcare provider can offer diagnosis and treatment plans tailored to the specifics of your condition, potentially mitigating further hair loss.

For children and teenagers experiencing hair loss, it's especially important to seek medical advice promptly. Hair loss at a young age can be particularly distressing and may be a sign of an autoimmune disorder or other health conditions. Professional guidance will not only address the physical aspects of the condition but can also provide support for dealing with its emotional impact.

In conclusion, if you're experiencing unexplained, sudden, or significant hair loss, it's wise not to wait. Consulting with a healthcare professional can offer you a clear diagnosis, peace of mind, and a pathway to treatment. Remember, the earlier you seek advice, the more options there may be available to you for managing and potentially reversing your hair loss.

CHAPTER 3
HOW DO I KNOW IF I HAVE ALOPECIA?

Realizing you might be experiencing alopecia can be an unsettling thought. After covering the basics of alopecia and its symptoms in the previous chapters, you might be wondering, "How do I confirm if what I'm experiencing is indeed alopecia?" This chapter aims to guide you through the diagnostic approaches and the logical next steps after suspecting that you might have alopecia. The journey to diagnosis is crucial, as it sets the stage for understanding your condition better and exploring treatment options.

First and foremost, if you've noticed significant hair loss or bald patches, it's time to consult a healthcare professional. Doctors usually start with a thorough medical history and physical examination. They'll want to understand the pattern of your hair loss, any family history of alopecia, and any other symptoms you might be experiencing. It's important to be as open and detailed as possible during these discussions, as it can significantly influence the diagnostic process.

Following the initial consultation, your doctor might suggest specific tests to rule out other causes of hair loss and confirm a diagnosis of alopecia. These tests can include blood tests to check for thyroid issues or nutritional deficiencies, scalp biopsies to examine the hair follicles, and pull tests to see how easily hair comes out. Each test provides valuable insights, helping to tailor a treatment plan that best suits your condition.

Another crucial aspect of diagnosing alopecia involves understanding the type you might be experiencing. With several forms of alopecia, ranging from Alopecia Areata, a condition where the immune system attacks hair follicles, to Androgenetic Alopecia, a patterned hair loss commonly associated with hormonal changes, the treatment and outlook can vary significantly. Identifying the specific type is a pivotal step in your alopecia journey, shaping the direction of subsequent treatments and interventions.

After the diagnosis, the next steps include exploring treatment options, which we'll discuss in the coming chapters. It's essential to approach this journey with patience and an open mind. Every individual's experience with alopecia is unique, and so is the path to managing it. The focus now shifts to understanding the causes in-depth and the multitude of treatments available. Armed with knowledge and support, navigating alopecia becomes a more manageable endeavor.

Diagnostic Approaches

Getting to the heart of whether or not you have alopecia can seem, at first glance, like walking through a maze without a map. However, medical science has come a long way in developing structured approaches to diagnose this condition accurately. It all begins with understanding the various ways professionals can pinpoint the cause and type of hair loss you're experiencing.

Initially, the journey often starts at your dermatologist's or trichologists office. These specialists are trained to recognize the signs of alopecia and can guide you through the first stages of diagnosis. The process typically kicks off with a detailed conversation about your medical history. Here, it's crucial to mention any family history of hair loss, recent stressful events, dietary habits, and any other health issues you might be facing. This broader look at your health can offer key insights since alopecia isn't just about what's happening on your head—it's often intertwined with your overall well-being.

After digging into your history, a physical examination is next. Your doctor or trichologist will take a close look at the pattern of your hair loss, checking for signs of natural thinning versus patchy, circular areas which are common signs of certain types of alopecia. Sometimes, they might also pull gently on a few strands of hair to see how easily they come out; an act known as the pull test. While it might seem simple, this test can provide valuable information about the stage and nature of your hair loss.

In some cases, a more thorough investigation is needed, and that's where scalp biopsies come in. This minor procedure involves taking a small sample of scalp skin and sending it to a lab for examination. Under the microscope, experts can identify patterns of hair loss, inflammation, and other factors that could be causing your alopecia. It might sound daunting, but it's a quick and typically pain-free way to get answers.

Blood tests to play a pivotal role in diagnosing alopecia, especially when there's a suspicion that it's linked to autoimmune diseases or nutritional deficiencies. Routine screenings can reveal issues like thyroid disease, low iron levels, or lupus, all of which can contribute to hair loss. By addressing these underlying conditions, oftentimes, the hair loss can be managed or even reversed.

Another tool in the diagnostic arsenal is trichoscopy, a non-invasive method that involves examining the scalp and hair using a specialized, handheld microscope called a dermatoscope. This technology offers a magnified view, enabling the doctor or trichologist to see details that are not visible to the naked eye. It's particularly effective in identifying the early signs of scarring alopecia and can also help in distinguishing between different types of alopecia.

If you're sitting in your dermatologist's or trichologists office wondering about the next steps, don't hesitate to ask about the diagnostic tests available. Understanding the methods used to diagnose alopecia can demystify the process and set your mind at ease. It's also a great way to become an active participant in your own healthcare journey.

Once the diagnostic process is underway, patience becomes an essential virtue. Some tests, like blood work or scalp biopsies, take time to yield results. It's important to stay in communication with your healthcare provider, keeping them informed about any changes in your condition or new symptoms that arise.

Finally, receiving a diagnosis of alopecia can be an emotional moment, but it's also a step towards understanding and managing your condition. With a clear diagnosis in hand, you and your healthcare team can tailor a treatment plan suited to your specific type of alopecia. Remember, the goal is not just to treat the symptoms but to ensure a healthier scalp and, ideally, hair regrowth.

In conclusion, the path to diagnosing alopecia involves a combination of personal medical history, physical examinations, and sometimes, more in-depth tests. Each step is designed to peel back the layers of uncertainty, offering clarity and a course of action. So, while the journey may initially feel overwhelming, know that there's a structured, science-backed pathway leading towards answers and, hopefully, successful management of alopecia.

The Next Step After My Diagnosis

Being diagnosed with alopecia can feel like being adrift in uncharted waters - it's both unexpected and life-altering. The initial shock and a myriad of emotions that follow are not only normal but also an integral part of your journey towards acceptance and management of the condition. The key question you might find yourself asking is, "What comes next?" This part of your journey is about transitioning from the uncertainty that accompanied seeking a diagnosis to a phase of proactive management and understanding of your condition.

After receiving your diagnosis, the next critical step involves developing a comprehensive treatment plan with your healthcare team. This plan is not a one-size-fits-all but rather a tailored approach that considers the specific type of alopecia you have, its severity, and your personal health history. Treatment options may range from medications and topical solutions to more advanced therapies. At this stage, it's vital to have open and honest discussions with your doctor about the potential benefits and side effects of each treatment option, allowing you to make informed decisions about your care.

Equally important is the need to educate yourself about alopecia. While your healthcare provider is a crucial resource, diving into credible sources and connecting with alopecia communities can offer additional support and insights. Understanding the underlying causes of alopecia, as discussed in subsequent chapters, not only demystifies the condition but also empowers you to advocate for your health effectively. Being well-informed can also mitigate the psychological impact of alopecia, paving the way for resilience and confidence despite the challenges.

Another aspect of navigating life post-diagnosis is addressing the emotional and psychological impacts. Alopecia is not just a physical condition; it's an experience that affects individuals deeply, touching on aspects of identity, self-esteem, and social interactions. Seeking support, whether through therapy, support groups, or conversations with loved ones, is essential. These resources not only provide a safe space to express and process your feelings but also introduce you to strategies for building a positive self-image and coping mechanisms for dealing with the societal pressures associated with hair loss.

Lastly, adopting healthy lifestyle choices can play a supportive role in managing alopecia. While there's no direct cure, maintaining a balanced diet, reducing stress, and avoiding triggers known to exacerbate hair loss can contribute to overall well-being and, in some cases, the management of symptoms. As we'll explore, nutrition and lifestyle modifications, though not a treatment per se, can create a conducive environment for managing the condition more effectively.

Tools and Tests Used by Professionals

When it comes to diagnosing and understanding alopecia, the tools and tests utilized by healthcare professionals are crucial. From physical assessments to cutting-edge technologies, these resources guide both diagnosis and treatment plans. Let's delve into the common techniques and tests that specialists use to confirm alopecia and its types.

One primary tool in the arsenal against alopecia is the clinical examination. This involves a thorough physical inspection of the scalp. Specialists look for patterns of hair loss, the condition of the scalp, and any signs of scarring alopecia. The presence of "exclamation mark" hairs, short hairs that taper at the base, can often be indicative of alopecia areata. This initial assessment can provide vital clues about the type of alopecia a person is experiencing.

Blood tests are another cornerstone of alopecia diagnosis. They are used to identify underlying conditions that might be causing hair loss, such as thyroid diseases, iron deficiency, or lupus. Specific tests can measure levels of hormones, iron stores, and markers of inflammation. Understanding the body's internal environment can often unlock answers as to why hair loss is occurring.

The pull test is a simple yet informative test. Here, a doctor gently pulls on a small section of hair to see how many hairs come out. This can help determine the severity of the hair loss and which stage of the growth cycle is affected. It's a direct method to assess if hair loss is active and how easily the hair is shed.

Scalp biopsy might sound intimidating, but it's a pivotal diagnostic tool. A small section of scalp skin, including hair follicles, is removed under local anesthesia and examined under a microscope. This can help identify the cause of hair loss, distinguishing between scarring and non-scarring forms. It's especially useful when the diagnosis isn't clear from other tests and examinations.

Dermoscopy, a technique involving a specialized magnifying tool, allows doctors to examine the scalp and hairs more closely. It's a non-invasive method that can identify patterns not visible to the naked eye, such as miniaturization of hair follicles in androgenetic alopecia or the dots and broken hairs characteristic of alopecia areata. Dermoscopy has become an indispensable tool in the dermatologist's kit for diagnosing different types of hair loss.

Trichoscopy, a form of dermoscopy specifically focused on the hair and scalp, can provide even more detailed insights. Through digital imagery and analysis, trichoscopy can evaluate hair shafts, measure their density, and assess the scalp's condition. It can be a key factor in monitoring the progression of one's alopecia over time and assessing the efficacy of treatments.

In certain cases, video microscopy is used to get an up-close look at the hair follicles and scalp. This tool can magnify the scalp up to 200 times, revealing details about hair shaft health and scalp condition. By examining these elements, professionals can provide tailored advice on treating and managing alopecia.

Finally, while not a diagnostic tool per se, genetic testing offers insights for some individuals. With advancements in science, genetic tests can identify markers associated with different types of alopecia, offering a glimpse into how genetics play a role in one's condition. This information can be crucial for understanding the likelihood of developing specific types of alopecia and tailoring prevention strategies accordingly.

In conclusion, the journey to diagnosing alopecia often involves a combination of these tools and tests. Each serve as a piece of the puzzle in understanding the full picture of one's hair loss. Through these advanced diagnostics, professionals can provide individuals with a clear diagnosis, empowering them with the knowledge to tackle their alopecia head-on.

CHAPTER 4
UNDERSTANDING ALOPECIA AND THE CAUSES

ALOPECIA, AS WE'VE ESTABLISHED IN THE PREVIOUS chapters, represents a complex condition that doesn't adhere to a single narrative. Journeying deeper into the heart of this condition, it's critical to unlock the door to its causes, which are as diverse as the condition itself. By delving into the science behind alopecia, we begin to see a clearer picture, where both genetics and the environment play pivotal roles.

At the genetic level, alopecia can sometimes run in families, suggesting a hereditary component. This doesn't mean that if a family member has alopecia, it's guaranteed that you'll experience the same, but it does increase the likelihood. On the flip side, alopecia isn't confined to genetic predispositions alone. Environmental triggers, such as extreme stress, hormonal changes, or exposure to certain chemicals, can contribute significantly. It paints a complex ecosystem where both inherent and external factors interplay, triggering alopecia in individuals.

Beyond the straightforward genetic and environmental triggers, there's a multitude of underlying causes that merit attention. Immune system irregularities, for instance, play a role in certain types of alopecia, where the body mistakenly attacks healthy hair follicles. This immune response underscores how alopecia is not just skin deep but is indicative of broader systemic issues. Moreover, lifestyle factors, including diet and stress management, hold potency in influencing hair health, demonstrating the condition's sensitivity to everyday habits and choices.

Understanding these causes offers not just clarity, but also empowerment. With knowledge comes the ability to navigate the alopecia journey with a sense of direction and control. It's crucial, however, to approach this information with a balanced perspective. While recognizing the role of genetics and environmental factors, it's also vital to remember that alopecia manifests uniquely in everyone. The same cause may not produce the same effect in different individuals, highlighting the importance of personalized approaches in managing this condition.

In summary, the story of alopecia is written not by a single author but by a chorus of genetic, environmental, and lifestyle factors. The causes of alopecia are as individual as the people it touches, requiring a nuanced understanding that respects the complexity of this condition. As we move forward, keeping an open mind and a proactive stance towards managing alopecia can pave the way for resilience and healing.

The Science Behind the Condition

Alopecia, often perceived merely as hair loss, unfolds as a tale far more intricate and multifaceted than initially meets the eye. At its core, alopecia represents a condition stemming from an amalgamation of factors that disrupt the normal cycle of hair growth. To truly grasp the essence of alopecia, it's imperative to delve into the biological and environmental components that orchestrate this condition.

First and foremost, hair growth occurs in a cycle that comprises three distinct phases: the anagen phase (growth phase), the catagen phase (transitional phase), and the telogen phase (resting phase). In a healthy individual, a majority of hair resides in the anagen phase, promoting continuous hair growth. However, in those afflicted with alopecia, this cycle undergoes a drastic alteration, often leading to premature termination of the anagen phase and a subsequent escalation in hair shedding.

The initiation of alopecia can be largely attributed to the immune system mistakenly targeting hair follicles. In autoimmune forms of alopecia, such as alopecia areata, the immune system perceives hair follicles as foreign invaders, akin to viruses or bacteria. This immune response culminates in inflammation around the follicles, thereby impeding their capacity to foster healthy hair growth.

Genetics also play a pivotal role in predisposing individuals to various types of alopecia. Research has identified specific genetic markers that are more prevalent in those with certain forms of alopecia, suggesting a hereditary component. This genetic predisposition does not guarantee the manifestation of alopecia but increases the likelihood of its occurrence, especially when combined with environmental triggers.

Environmental triggers, encompassing a broad spectrum of factors, can precipitate alopecia in genetically susceptible individuals. Such triggers include stress, hormonal changes, medications, and nutritional deficiencies, each capable of disrupting the hair growth cycle or exacerbating immune system activity against hair follicles.

Stress, both physical and emotional, has been recognized as a significant precipitator of alopecia. It can instigate a telogen effluvium, a condition where an increased number of hairs enter the telogen phase, culminating in noticeable hair shedding. This form of alopecia is typically transient and can be reversed by alleviating stress.

Hormonal fluctuations, particularly those associated with thyroid disorders, pregnancy, and menopause, have been implicated in various forms of alopecia. These hormonal changes can disrupt the equilibrium of the hair cycle, promoting hair loss or thinning.

Certain medications and treatments, such as chemotherapy, are known to induce alopecia by forcefully halting cellular division in hair follicles. This abrupt interruption of the hair growth cycle results in widespread hair loss, though it often reverses once the medication is discontinued.

Nutritional deficiencies, specifically in iron, zinc, and certain vitamins, can impair hair follicle nutrition, impeding their ability to sustain normal hair growth. Correcting these deficiencies often ameliorates hair health, underscoring the importance of a balanced diet.

Beyond individual factors, the interplay between genetics and the environment quintessentially underscores the complexity of alopecia. It's the convergence of these elements, each influencing hair growth in a distinct manner, that culminates in the onset of alopecia. Understanding this interplay is crucial for comprehending the multifaceted nature of the condition.

Furthermore, it's imperative to acknowledge the uniqueness of each alopecia case. While certain patterns and commonalities exist, the manifestation of alopecia can vary widely among individuals, influenced by their genetic makeup and environmental exposures. This variability underscores the need for personalized approaches in both diagnosis and treatment.

In exploring the science behind alopecia, researchers continue to unearth new insights into its etiology and pathogenesis. Advanced technologies and methodologies, from genetic sequencing to immunological studies, provide a deeper understanding of the mechanisms driving alopecia. These discoveries not only illuminate the complexity of the condition but also pave the way for novel therapeutic strategies.

The pursuit of understanding alopecia necessitates a holistic view, considering not only the biological aspects of the condition but also the environmental and psychological factors that contribute to its development. It's a condition that exemplifies the intricate interplay between our bodies and the world around us, emphasizing the need for a comprehensive approach in both study and care.

In essence, the science behind alopecia is a testament to the dynamic interplay of genetics, physiology, and environment. As we continue to unravel the mysteries of this condition, it's important to foster empathy and support for those navigating the challenges it presents. The journey toward understanding and managing alopecia is ongoing, and each discovery brings hope for more effective interventions and a deeper comprehension of the condition's complexities.

Genetic Factors

Genetic factors play a pivotal role in understanding alopecia, a hair loss condition that perplexes and troubles many. Diving into the genetics behind alopecia not only unpacks the hereditary aspects of this complex condition but also illuminates why some individuals are more predisposed to developing it than others. It's a fascinating journey into the weave of our DNA, where the story of alopecia and its relationship with our genes unfolds.

At its core, alopecia is not a one-size-fits-all condition. Its manifestation can range from the well-known pattern baldness, often seen in men, to more diffuse and widespread hair loss across the scalp and body. What intrigues scientists and medical professionals is the clear evidence pointing towards a hereditary link, especially in conditions like androgenetic alopecia, also known as male or female pattern baldness.

Research has shown that individuals with a family history of alopecia are at a higher risk of experiencing hair loss themselves. It's a matter of not if, but when for some, as their genetic makeup nudges them down a path, they've seen other family members walk. This genetic predisposition involves a multitude of genes, making it a polygenic condition. It's not about a single culprit but a consortium of genetic factors that play into the risk of developing alopecia.

One specific gene of interest in the study of androgenetic alopecia is the AR gene, which provides instructions for making a protein called an androgen receptor. Androgens are hormones that play a role in male traits and reproductive activity. They are also involved in regulating hair growth. The interaction between androgens and the androgen receptor gene can influence the risk of developing androgenetic alopecia, making some individuals more susceptible than others.

Furthermore, the complexity of alopecia's genetic basis is underscored by studies indicating the involvement of the 20p11 region of the chromosome in non-androgenetic forms of alopecia, such as alopecia areata. This autoimmune condition, which results in patchy hair loss, highlights the variety of ways genes can influence hair health and susceptibility to hair loss conditions.

Understanding the genetic makeup of alopecia is not merely an academic pursuit; it has practical implications for treatment and management. For individuals grappling with the condition, recognizing the genetic component offers a form of solace: their hair loss is not a result of something they've done but rather a prewritten script in their genetic code. This knowledge can shift the focus towards management and treatment options that consider their unique genetic backdrop.

Indeed, the identification of specific genes associated with alopecia has opened the door for genetic testing. These tests can assess an individual's risk of developing the condition, leading to early intervention strategies that might minimize the impact of hair loss. It's a proactive approach, arming individuals with information about their predisposition and allowing them to plan accordingly.

However, it's important to tread cautiously in the realm of genetic testing for alopecia. The multifactorial nature of the condition means that genetics is just one piece of the puzzle. Environmental factors, lifestyle, and hormonal fluctuations also play significant roles. Thus, a genetic predisposition does not guarantee the development of alopecia, just as the absence of a known genetic risk does not assure immunity from the condition.

The potential for tailored treatments based on an individual's genetic profile is on the horizon. As research delves deeper into the specific genetic markers associated with different forms of alopecia, the prospect of personalized medicine becomes more promising. This could mean treatments that are more effective, with minimal side effects, targeted to an individual's genetic makeup.

Yet, the interplay between genes and the environment complicates the picture. It's a dynamic dance where genes set the stage, but lifestyle and environmental factors cue in the music. Recognizing this intricate relationship is crucial in adopting a holistic approach to treating and managing alopecia. It's not solely about altering one's genetic destiny but also about modifying what we can control — our environment, lifestyle, and stress levels.

One can't talk about genetic factors without touching upon the emotional and psychological impact. Knowing that one's hair loss is influenced by genetics can elicit a range of emotions, from relief at having an explanation to frustration over the lack of control. This underscores the importance of psychological support and counseling for individuals dealing with alopecia. Acceptance and understanding of the condition, within the framework of genetic predisposition, can be a significant step in coping with hair loss.

In families where alopecia is a common thread, conversations about the genetic aspects can foster a supportive environment. Sharing experiences and knowledge about the hereditary nature of alopecia can prepare younger members for potential outcomes, while also underscoring the importance of early intervention and management strategies. It's about passing down knowledge, alongside genes, to empower future generations.

Fundamentally, the journey into the genetics of alopecia is far from over. As advances in genetic research continue, the hope for unlocking further secrets of alopecia lies on the horizon. These discoveries not only promise more effective treatments but also a deeper understanding of the condition. It's a step towards demystifying alopecia, reframing it not as a condition of loss but as one of understanding, management, and hope.

In conclusion, the genetic factors underlying alopecia offer both challenges and opportunities. While the hereditary nature of alopecia can make it seem like an inevitable journey for some, advancements in genetics and medicine are paving the way for more personalized and effective interventions. The exploration of our genetic codes is leading us towards a future where managing alopecia is not just about treating symptoms but understanding and addressing its roots in our DNA. This, combined with a compassionate approach that acknowledges the emotional impact of hair loss, holds the key to a more hopeful narrative for individuals affected by alopecia.

Environmental Triggers

Environmental Triggers can significantly contribute to the onset and progression of alopecia, a condition that results in hair loss and can dramatically impact an individual's quality of life. As we navigate through the complexities of this condition, understanding the interplay between our environment and our health becomes crucial. Various environmental factors, ranging from pollutants to lifestyle choices, play a pivotal role in exacerbating or potentially triggering alopecia in susceptible individuals.

Firstly, exposure to certain chemicals and pollutants has been implicated in the development of alopecia. Studies suggest that airborne pollutants, including smoke and industrial emissions, can contribute to scalp irritation and inflammation, leading to or worsening hair loss. These pollutants can create oxidative stress on scalp follicles, depriving them of necessary nutrients and leading to the deterioration of hair health. Additionally, heavy metals found in water supplies, such as lead and arsenic, have also been associated with increased risk of alopecia, highlighting the importance of environmental safety and regulation.

Secondly, lifestyle factors, including stress and diet, operate as significant environmental triggers. High stress levels, often resultant of our fast-paced, modern lifestyle, can lead to a type of hair loss known as telogen effluvium. This condition forces hair follicles into a resting phase, causing hair to thin and fall out prematurely. Similarly, diets lacking in essential nutrients, vitamins, and minerals crucial for hair growth and scalp health can exacerbate hair loss. This connection underscores the importance of a balanced diet and stress management as preventive measures against alopecia.

Furthermore, seasonal changes and exposure to sunlight have also been observed to influence alopecia. Seasonal fluctuations, particularly extreme changes in temperature, can affect the hair growth cycle, potentially leading to increased shedding during certain times of the year. While moderate exposure to sunlight is beneficial for vitamin D synthesis, essential for healthy hair follicles, excessive UV exposure can damage the scalp and hair, again emphasizing the delicate balance our body requires with its environment.

In conclusion, while the genetic predisposition to alopecia cannot be altered, understanding and mitigating environmental triggers is within our grasp. By adopting a lifestyle that minimizes exposure to harmful pollutants, manages stress, and ensures a nutrient-rich diet, individuals can potentially reduce their risk of developing alopecia or lessen its severity. This holistic approach to managing alopecia not only addresses the physical aspects of hair loss but also contributes to overall well-being, making it a critical component of alopecia management strategies.

41

CHAPTER 5
THE PSYCHOLOGICAL IMPACT OF ALOPECIA

ALOPECIA, WHILE PREDOMINANTLY RECOGNIZED AS A physical condition, casts a deep shadow over the psychological well-being of those it touches. The sudden or gradual loss of hair can trigger a profound transformation in how individuals perceive themselves and are perceived by the world. This chapter delves into the myriad ways alopecia can impact mental health, and importantly, strategies to navigate these turbulent waters. The journey of coming to terms with alopecia is as much an inward one as it is about external adaptation.

First and foremost, the initial diagnosis of alopecia can elicit a spectrum of emotional responses – shock, denial, anger, and grief are common. It's a disruption of one's identity and body image, areas deeply intertwined with our self-esteem and confidence. The societal emphasis on hair as a symbol of beauty and vitality only magnifies these feelings, leading to increased stress and, in some cases, social withdrawal. It's crucial to acknowledge these emotions as valid and integral to the healing process.

Beyond the immediate emotional turbulence, alopecia can usher in long-term psychological challenges. Anxiety and depression are frequently reported, fueled by persistent worries over the unpredictability of hair loss and its visibility to others. The fear of public judgment or ridicule can be paralyzing, urging a reevaluation of public engagements and relationships. This period demands a compassionate understanding from peers and society, fostering a supportive environment where individuals feel seen beyond their hair loss.

However, amidst these challenges, there lies an opportunity for profound personal growth and resilience. Many find strength in community—connecting with others facing similar trials through support groups, forums, and social media channels. These platforms offer not just solace, but shared knowledge and strategies for embracing one's appearance. The act of sharing one's story can be incredibly empowering, turning a narrative of loss into one of defiance and acceptance.

Building resilience and confidence in the face of alopecia is no small feat, yet it is undeniably possible. It often involves redefining personal beauty standards, embracing creative expressions of identity such as fashion and accessories, and, importantly, practicing self-compassion. Psychological counseling and therapy can also play a pivotal role in navigating this journey, providing tools to manage negative thoughts and foster a positive self-image. As we move forward, understanding and addressing the psychological impact of alopecia is paramount in ensuring that individuals don't just cope, but thrive.

Dealing with Emotional Well-Being

When grappling with alopecia, the focus often leans heavily towards the physical manifestations of the condition, putting the substantial psychological impact on the back burner. The journey through alopecia isn't just about the absence of hair; it's deeply intertwined with the psychological well-being of an individual. The sudden or gradual loss can trigger a cascade of emotional responses, from shock and embarrassment to profound sadness and anxiety. In this section, we'll navigate through the emotional terrain that accompanies alopecia and explore ways to nurture mental and emotional health.

Understanding the emotional rollercoaster that comes with alopecia is the first step to managing it. It's common to experience a blow to one's self-esteem and self-image, feelings that are profoundly personal and can affect every aspect of life. The social and cultural significance attached to hair makes coping with its loss all the more challenging. Many people report feeling exposed or naked without their natural hair, leading to social withdrawal or avoiding situations where their condition might be noticed. Acknowledging these feelings is crucial to the healing process, validating that it's not just "hair" but a significant part of your identity.

Building resilience and finding confidence in your identity beyond your physical appearance is a journey worth embarking upon. It involves redefining personal beauty standards and embracing the new self with acceptance and compassion. Organizations and support groups play a pivotal role in this aspect, providing a platform for sharing experiences and coping strategies. Hearing stories from others who've walked a similar path can be incredibly comforting, offering hope and solidarity. Moreover, professional counseling or therapy can provide tailored strategies to manage negative emotions and rebuild self-esteem.

Engaging in activities that promote mental and physical wellness is another avenue to support emotional well-being. Exercise, meditation, and pursuing hobbies encourage positive mental health and provide a distraction from the relentless focus on hair loss. It's also helpful to connect with friends and family, talking openly about your feelings and experiences. Such connections often bring a different perspective, high-lighting attributes and strengths overshadowed by the struggles with alopecia.

In conclusion, while the journey with alopecia can be fraught with emotional turmoil, there's a pathway to resilience and acceptance. The significance of addressing and nurturing emotional well-being cannot be over-stated. By understanding the emotional impact, seeking support, and embracing a holistic approach to wellness, individuals can find a way to thrive despite their condi-tion. Alopecia might alter the way you look, but it doesn't define who you are or your value as a person. Embracing this mindset is key to not just coping but living fully with alopecia.

Building Resilience and Confidence

While managing the physical aspects of alopecia is crucial, tending to your emotional well-being is equally important. Alopecia, though not physically painful, can take a significant toll on one's mental health, affecting self-esteem and confidence. However, building resilience can empower you to navigate this journey with strength and grace. This section provides strategies to bolster your confidence and resilience, ensuring you're equipped to face the challenges that come with alopecia.

First and foremost, understanding that your self-worth is not tied to your appearance is vital. It's easier said than done, especially in a society that often prioritizes external beauty. However, shifting focus to qualities that define your character—like your courage, kindness, and intelligence—can help you build a foundation of self-esteem that extends beyond the physical. Engaging in activities and hobbies that reinforce these aspects of your identity can also fortify your sense of self and contribute to overall well-being.

Another key aspect is fostering a supportive community. Surrounding yourself with people who understand and empathize with your experience can make a significant difference. Support groups, either in-person or online, provide a space to share stories, advice, and encouragement. Learning from others who are on a similar path can offer valuable insights and remind you that you're not alone. These communities can also be a great resource for practical tips on dealing with the day-to-day aspects of living with alopecia.

Practicing self-care is another fundamental way to build resilience. This might include regular exercise, which not only improves physical health but can boost mood and reduce stress. Mindfulness practices, such as meditation and deep breathing exercises, can also help manage anxiety and foster a positive mindset. Moreover, exploring creative outlets like writing, art, or music can be therapeutic, providing a means to express your feelings and process your experiences.

Lastly, consider seeking professional help if you find it challenging to cope with the emotional impact of alopecia. Therapists or counselors specialized in dealing with chronic conditions or body image issues can offer personalized strategies to build confidence and resilience. Remember, reaching out for support is a sign of strength, not weakness. By prioritizing both your physical and emotional well-being, you can navigate alopecia with confidence, embracing the journey with resilience and optimism.

CHAPTER 6
MEDICATIONS AND TOPICAL SOLUTIONS

As we strive deeper into the exploration of treatments for alopecia, we uncover a realm of potential solutions. The journey for individuals facing hair loss is deeply personal and varies significantly from one person to the next. Medications and topical solutions stand as a beacon of hope, offering a chance to regain not only hair but also a sense of normalcy and self-confidence. Let's explore the pharmaceutical and topical options available that have shown promise in the battle against alopecia.

First on the list are corticosteroids, powerful anti-inflammatory drugs that can help tame the autoimmune response thought to be a key player in alopecia areata. These medications are available in various forms, including injectable, oral, and topical. The injectable form, directly administered into the scalp, has been heralded for its effectiveness in prompting hair regrowth in localized areas. Oral corticosteroids, while potent, are generally considered a last resort due to their wide array of side effects. Topical corticosteroids, meanwhile, are easier to apply and carry a lower risk of systemic side effects, making them a preferred choice for many.

Minoxidil, a topical treatment better known by its brand name Rogaine, is another frontline defense against hair loss. Originally developed as a treatment for high blood pressure, Minoxidil's hair regrowth properties were discovered almost by chance. It works by widening blood vessels, which in turn improves blood flow to the hair follicles. This over-the-counter solution requires consistent application, and while results can vary, it has offered a glimmer of hope to many grappling with alopecia.

For those navigating the turbulent waters of more severe forms of alopecia, such as alopecia totalis and alopecia universalis, newer treatments like Janus kinase (JAK) inhibitors are on the horizon. These powerful drugs, still undergoing clinical trials for hair loss, target specific pathways in the immune system. Early results are promising, showing potential for significant hair regrowth in individuals who have not responded well to other treatments.

Topical immunotherapy is another avenue being

explored, especially for those with extensive alopecia areata. This treatment involves deliberately inducing an allergic reaction on the scalp with chemicals such as diphencyprone (DPCP) or squaric acid dibutylester (SADBE). The theory here is to distract the immune system away from attacking hair follicles and instead, mobilize it against the induced allergen. This method has shown success in stimulating hair growth in some patients, albeit with the downside of having to induce an allergic reaction.

It's also important to mention the role of anthralin, a synthetic, tar-like substance that is applied topically. Anthralin is designed to alter the skin's immune function, thereby encouraging hair regrowth. Despite its potential messiness and the need for careful application to avoid skin irritation, anthralin can be an effective option for some individuals with alopecia areata.

Finasteride, known by its brand name Propecia, is a medication more commonly prescribed for androgenetic alopecia, or pattern hair loss. It works by inhibiting the production of dihydrotestosterone (DHT), a hormone linked to hair loss in men. While finasteride has proven effective in many cases, it's used predominantly in male patients due to its potential side effects in women, especially those of childbearing age.

When considering these medications and topical solutions, it's crucial to consult with a healthcare professional. They can provide guidance tailored to your specific condition and help navigate the potential side effects and benefits. It's also worth noting that patience is key; many of these treatments require time to show results, and the journey to hair regrowth is often a marathon, not a sprint.

As we continue to explore treatments for alopecia, it's paramount to remember that each individual's journey is unique. What works for one person may not work for another, underscoring the importance of a personalized approach to treatment. In the following sections, we'll delve deeper into alternative and emerging therapies, as well as the role of diet and supplements in managing alopecia, building upon our foundation with a holistic view of treatment options.

In conclusion, the landscape of medications and topical solutions for alopecia is rich and varied, offering numerous paths toward potential regrowth and recovery. As research advances and new treatments emerge, there's a growing sense of hope for individuals affected by alopecia. Armed with knowledge and the support of the medical community, navigating the journey of hair loss can become a testament to resilience and the pursuit of well-being.

Alternative and Emerging Therapies

As we explore the realm of treatments available for those dealing with alopecia, it's imperative to recognize the innovative and non-traditional therapies that are gaining attention. In recent years, the focus has shifted not only to addressing the symptoms but also to understanding and treating the underlying causes of hair loss. This shift has brought forth various alternative and emerging therapies that promise new hope for individuals seeking solutions outside the conventional scope of medications and topical treatments.

Among these emerging therapies, the use of low-level laser therapy (LLLT) is noteworthy. This method employs the use of specific wavelengths of light to stimulate hair growth at the cellular level. It's a non-invasive option that has shown promising results in clinical trials, offering a ray of hope for many who haven't found success with traditional treatments. The appeal of LLLT lies in its simplicity and the absence of significant side effects, marking it as a favorable choice for many seeking new avenues of treatment.

Another area of interest is the use of platelet-rich plasma (PRP) injections. This procedure involves drawing a patient's blood, processing it to enrich the platelets, and then injecting it into the scalp. The concentrated platelets release growth factors that are thought to stimulate hair regrowth and healing. While still under research, PRP injections have garnered attention for their potential to improve hair density without the need for daily medication or topical application.

A look into the horizon also reveals the exploration of stem cell therapy as a novel approach to combatting alopecia. This cutting-edge therapy aims to regenerate or repair damaged hair follicles, offering a potentially permanent solution to hair loss. The process involves taking stem cells from the patient or a donor and administering them into the scalp region where hair growth is desired. Though still in the experimental phase, the promise of stem cell therapy ignites optimism among both patients and researchers for its revolutionary approach to treating hair loss.

As the landscape of alopecia treatment continues to evolve, it's clear that the journey doesn't end with the traditional methods we've come to know. The emergence of these alternative therapies opens up a world of potential for individuals seeking to reclaim not only their hair but also their confidence and sense of normalcy. While these treatments offer great promise, it's important for individuals to consult with healthcare professionals to understand the best course of action for their specific situation. The path to managing alopecia is as diverse as the individuals it affects, and with continuous research and innovation, the future looks hopeful for finding more effective and long-lasting solutions.

The Role of Diet and Supplements

As we navigate through the complexities of alopecia, it's crucial to explore the contribution of diet and supplements in managing this condition. While medications and topical solutions often take center stage in treatment plans, the significance of nutritional support should not be underestimated.

First and foremost, it's important to acknowledge that a well-balanced diet plays a foundational role in hair health. Nutritional deficiencies can exacerbate hair loss, making it imperative for individuals with alopecia to focus on nutrient-rich foods. For example, proteins are the building blocks of hair, as hair follicles are made mostly of protein. A lack of adequate protein in the diet can, therefore, contribute to hair loss.

Iron is another critical nutrient. It helps red blood cells carry oxygen to your cells, including hair follicles, and deficiencies in iron can lead to hair loss or exacerbate alopecia symptoms. Foods rich in iron, such as spinach, lean meats, and legumes, should be integral parts of your diet.

Zinc plays a role in hair tissue growth and repair. It also helps keep the oil glands around the follicles working properly. Hair loss is a common symptom of zinc deficiency. Thus, incorporating foods like oysters, beef, and pumpkin seeds, which are high in zinc, can be beneficial.

Vitamin D deficiency has been linked to alopecia areata and may play a role in other forms of alopecia as well. Spending time in sunlight can help your body produce Vitamin D, but it's also found in foods like fatty fish, mushrooms, and fortified products.

In addition to these nutrients, omega-3 and omega-6 fatty acids have been shown to improve hair density and decrease hair loss when taken as supplements. These healthy fats, found in fish oil, flaxseeds, and walnuts, among other foods, can enhance the health of your scalp and hair.

Beyond individual nutrients, the overall quality of your diet matters. Diets high in processed foods and sugar can contribute to inflammation, which is associated with an increased risk of alopecia. Shifting towards a Mediterranean diet, rich in fruits, vegetables, whole grains, and healthy fats, can support overall health and potentially improve hair health.

Supplements can also play a significant role, especially for individuals unable to meet their nutritional needs through diet alone. Biotin, a B-vitamin known for its role in hair health, is commonly recommended.

However, it's crucial to discuss with a healthcare professional before starting any new supplement, as excessive intake of certain nutrients can have adverse effects.

Antioxidants, including vitamins E and C, can combat oxidative stress which may contribute to alopecia. There's emerging evidence suggesting that antioxidants might play a role in managing alopecia by protecting hair follicles from damage.

In conclusion, while diet and supplements are not a cure-all for alopecia, they play a pivotal role in supporting hair health and potentially alleviating some symptoms of the condition. Creating a well-rounded diet that emphasizes nutrient-dense foods, along with targeted supplementation under the guidance of a healthcare provider, can form an integral part of managing alopecia.

CHAPTER 7
HEALTHY CHOICES

After understanding the complexity of alopecia, from its varying types to the psychological toll it can take, it's crucial to emphasize lifestyle habits that bolster overall well-being. Embarking on a journey to make healthier choices can be transformative, especially in managing conditions like alopecia. These alternatives don't just center on physical health but also encompass mental and emotional resilience, essential components in navigating this condition.

Maintaining a balanced diet, engaging in regular physical activity, and ensuring adequate sleep are foundational elements of a healthy lifestyle. For individuals coping with alopecia, these practices might seem peripheral but they're integral to managing the condition effectively. A well-nourished body is better equipped to handle stress, which in turn, may reduce the severity or frequency of alopecia flare-ups. Exercise, too, plays a critical role by enhancing blood circulation, potentially benefiting scalp health and promoting hair strength.

Beyond the physical, mental well-being is paramount. Stress is both a potential trigger and consequence of alopecia, creating a cycle that can exacerbate the condition. Incorporating stress-reduction techniques such as mindfulness, meditation, or yoga can be pivotal. These practices not only diminish stress levels but also improve one's relationship with their body and hair, fostering a positive self-image. Embracing supportive communities—whether online or in person—provides an additional layer of emotional sustenance, reinforcing the fact that one is not navigating this path alone.

Environmental choices also have a role to play. Reducing exposure to harsh chemicals, whether in hair care products or daily environments, can minimize potential irritants that may worsen alopecia. Opting for gentle, natural hair care routines and being cautious about physical stressors on the hair and scalp can be beneficial preventative measures. These adaptations, while seemingly minor, contribute to a holistic approach to managing alopecia.

Ultimately, the journey through alopecia is deeply personal yet undeniably influenced by an array of lifestyle factors. Making concerted efforts to choose healthily across various aspects of life may offer some control and empowerment in an otherwise unpredictable condition. A series of healthy choices can significantly enhance the quality of life.

CHAPTER 8
THE ROLE OF NUTRITION IN MANAGING ALOPECIA

Moving on from the foundational understanding and emotional impacts associated with alopecia, it's time to dive into an often-overlooked aspect of managing this condition: nutrition. The food we consume plays a crucial yet subtle role in maintaining the health of our hair. It's not just about eating for energy or controlling weight; it's about feeding the follicles with the right nutrients to support hair growth and resilience.

Nutrient deficiencies are known culprits in the tale of hair loss. For instance, low levels of iron, zinc, and vitamins D and B12 can intensify or even trigger alopecia. This isn't to say that popping a bunch of supplements is a magic cure for hair loss, but it does underscore the importance of a balanced diet. Incorporating a diverse array of foods can help ensure that your body gets the wide range of vitamins and minerals it needs to keep your hair on your head. Foods rich in omega-3 fatty acids, protein, and antioxidants can particularly offer support to those battling alopecia, nourishing the scalp and potentially reducing inflammation that might contribute to hair loss.

However, navigating nutrition for alopecia isn't just about what to add to your diet; it's also about noting what to limit. Foods that may trigger inflammation or hormonal imbalances, for some people, can exacerbate hair loss. Everyone's body reacts differently, but being mindful of how certain foods affect you personally is a critical piece of the puzzle. An elimination diet, guided by a healthcare professional, can sometimes reveal if certain foods are contributing to your alopecia.

Given the intricate ties between diet and hair health, it's not surprising that different cultures have developed unique dietary approaches to combat alopecia. From the use of specific herbs and spices lauded for their hair benefits in traditional Indian medicine to the Mediterranean diet's emphasis on fresh, antioxidant-rich foods, there are global wisdoms to glean from. These international practices underscore the universal quest for health and well-being, extending beyond alopecia management to foster overall vitality.

Critically, while nutrition is a powerful tool in the battle against alopecia, it's crucial to view it as part of a holistic approach to management. Proper nutrition can support and enhance other treatments, but it's not usually a standalone solution. Regular consultation with health-care providers, combined with personalized dietary strategies, can pave the most effective path forward for individuals dealing with alopecia. Remember, your diet is another part of your arsenal in maintaining your health, resilience, and well-being in the face of alopecia.

How Your Diet Influences Hair Health

As we look into the role of nutrition in managing alopecia, it's crucial to understand how profoundly your diet can influence the health of your hair. Nutrition isn't just about weight management or heart health; it has a direct connection to the vitality, strength, and even the growth cycle of your hair. Just as every plant needs the right nutrients to flourish, your hair requires specific vitamins and minerals to grow and remain strong.

First and foremost, protein plays a vital role in hair health. Hair is primarily made of keratin, a type of protein. A diet lacking in adequate protein can lead to weak, brittle hair, and in severe cases, it can contribute to hair loss. Including sources of lean protein in your diet, such as fish, poultry, eggs, and legumes, can support the building blocks of hair.

Iron is another cornerstone nutrient for hair. It helps red blood cells carry oxygen to your cells, including those that stimulate hair growth. Low levels of iron, which can result in anemia, are a well-documented cause of hair loss. Incorporating iron-rich foods like spinach, lentils, and red meat into your meals can help prevent deficiency. For those who prefer not to consume meat, consider pairing plant-based iron sources with vitamin C-rich foods to enhance absorption.

Omega-3 fatty acids are known for their anti-inflammatory properties, aiding in opening up the hair follicles and promoting hair growth. These essential fats, found in fish like salmon, sardines, and mackerel, as well as in flaxseeds and walnuts, can't be produced by the body and must be obtained through diet. They not only encourage hair growth but also add elasticity to your hair, preventing it from breaking.

Vitamins such as biotin, zinc, and vitamins A, E, and D also play significant roles in hair health. Biotin, for example, is often touted for its ability to strengthen hair and nails. While deficiencies in these vitamins and minerals are not the sole cause of alopecia, ensuring your diet is rich in these nutrients can contribute to healthier hair. Fruits, vegetables, nuts, and seeds are excellent sources of these vital nutrients. Given the intricate relationship between diet and hair health, making mindful dietary choices can be a powerful way to manage alopecia. While it may not cure the condition, incorporating a balanced diet rich in key nutrients can certainly help in minimizing hair loss and promoting the growth of healthy hair.

Cultural Insights and International Approaches to Treatment

Nutrition plays a critical role in the management of alopecia across different cultures and countries, presenting a multitude of beliefs, remedies, and diet-based solutions tailored to combat hair loss. It's fascinating to observe how various international approaches and cultural insights contribute to our understanding and treatment of alopecia. Across the globe, dietary approaches to managing this condition are as diverse as they are insightful, offering a unique perspective on the universal quest for health and well-being.

In Mediterranean regions, for instance, the diet is rich in omega-3 fatty acids, antioxidants, and polyphenols, largely owing to the consumption of olive oil, fresh fruits, and vegetables. This diet is heralded not only for its heart health benefits but also for its potential to strengthen hair follicles and prevent hair loss. On the other hand, in East Asian countries, diets high in fermented foods and seafood provide a different set of nutrients like selenium and B vitamins, which are key for maintaining scalp health and hair integrity.

Looking further, traditional Indian medicine, known as Ayurveda, offers a holistic approach to alopecia, emphasizing a balanced diet alongside herbal treatments. Foods that balance the "pitta" dosha, which is believed to cause hair loss when in excess, are encouraged. These include cooling and nourishing foods like green leafy vegetables, aloe vera, and nuts. Ayurvedic practices also recommend specific herbs and spices, such as Brahmi and Amla, known for their hair rejuvenating properties.

In contrast, Western approaches often lean towards a more scientific methodology, highlighting the importance of vitamins and minerals such as biotin, zinc, and iron in diet supplements. The influence of the Mediterranean diet has also permeated western cultures, acknowledging the impact of a balanced diet on overall health, including that of hair. Additionally, the rise of holistic wellness in Western societies has seen a blend of Eastern dietary practices being adopted, such as the inclusion of fermented foods and herbal supplements into daily diets.

What becomes clear is that while the specifics of dietary recommendations may vary from culture to culture, the underlying principle remains consistent: nutrition is a foundational element in the fight against alopecia. The international mosaic of dietary practices enriches our understanding and approach to managing this condition, emphasizing that a well-rounded, nutrient-rich diet is beneficial, no matter where you are in the world. It's a testament to the idea that sometimes, the best way forward is by looking at the wisdom of those who've come before us, from all corners of the globe.

Before and After Treatment

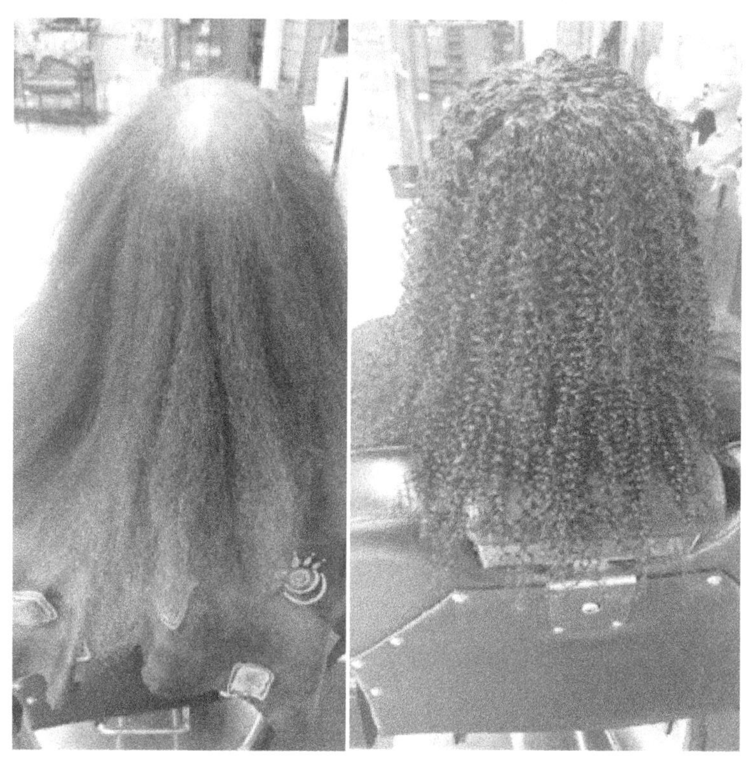

Before and After Treatment

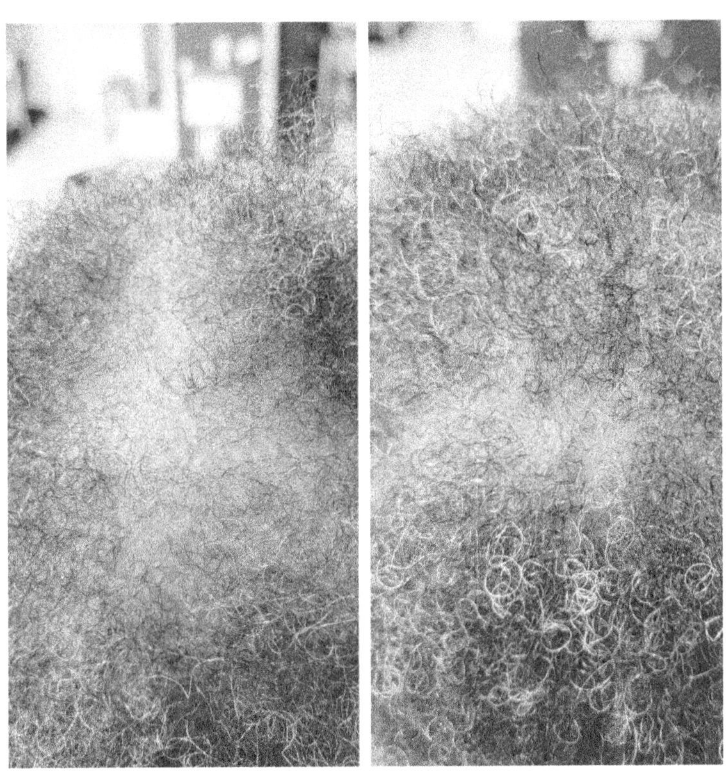

AFTERWORD

As we close the chapter on our journey through understanding alopecia, it's crucial to reflect on the crucial insights we've uncovered. Alopecia, with its multitude of forms and triggers, isn't just a condition that affects the scalp but is deeply interwoven with every aspect of an individual's life, from their self-image to how they interact with the world. Through an exploration of its symptoms, causes, and the innovative treatments available, we've researched deep into what makes alopecia such a unique condition to confront.

Tackling alopecia head-on isn't solely about medical interventions or dietary changes, although these play significant roles. It's also about nurturing resilience, embracing support from within one's community, and understanding that while alopecia might be a part of one's life, it doesn't define who they are. We've seen how emotional well-being is just as critical as physical health in managing alopecia and why building a support network, including healthcare professionals, family, and friends, can be incredibly empowering.

In essence, the fight against alopecia is multifaceted, involving a blend of science, and personal courage. As you move forward, remember that every journey is personal and unique. What works for one might not work for another, and that's okay. The most important takeaway is to keep exploring, keep learning, and never lose hope. With each passing day, we're getting closer to more understanding, better treatments, and, ultimately, a world where alopecia's impact on lives can be minimized.